Overcoming Lupus Handbook:

Detailed Guide on How to Overcome Lupus, How to Carry Out Its diagnosis & Its Treatment as Well as Other Reliable Remedies

By

Dr. Geraldine E. Oneal

Copyright@2020

TABLE OF CONTENTS

CHAPTER ONE...3

    LUPUS DEFINITION 3

CHAPTER TWO...7

    THE TYPES OF LUPUS..........................7

CHAPTER THREE 11

    SYMPTOMS OF LUPUS THAT ARE
    KNOWN 11

CHAPTER FOUR..22

    REAL CAUSES OF LUPUS 22

CHAPTER FIVE..27

    EFFICIENT DIAGNOSIS OF LUPUS.......27

CHAPTER SIX..35

    TREATING LUPUS QUICKLY AND
    EFFECTIVELY 35

The End...51

CHAPTER ONE

LUPUS DEFINITION

Lupus is as it is called is essentially a foundational immune system illness or ailment that happens at whatever point the safe arrangement of the human body assaults its own tissues just as organs in the body.

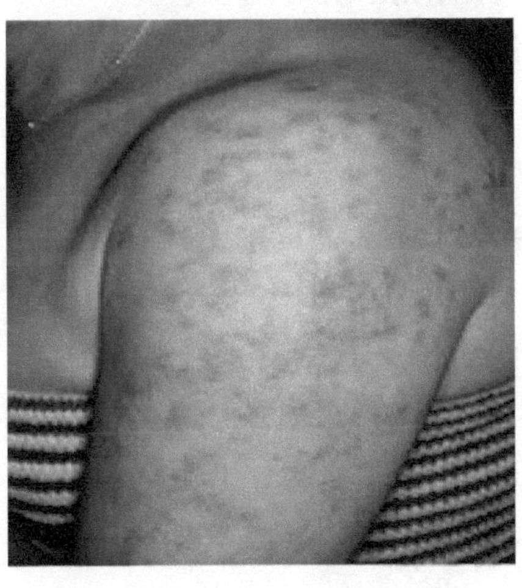

Furthermore, aggravation
that is brought about by
lupus could truly influence a
scope of body frameworks
including heart, cerebrum,
lungs, platelets, kidneys,
skin just as joints.

Additionally, lupus can be
intricate to analyze just in
light of the fact that the signs
just as the side effects look
like those of different
afflictions or illnesses.

Especially, the most widely
recognized indication of
lupus is a remarkable rash
that takes after the wings of
butterflies unfurling over the
two cheeks, and it shows up

in practically all occurrences or instances of lupus.

In addition, a few people are brought into the world with the affinity to have lupus while it might likewise be realized by the accompanying:

*Infections

*Drugs

*Sunlight

Discover more in the following parts as I accept

you through the astonishing
just as enduring methods of
disposing of lupus.

CHAPTER TWO

THE TYPES OF LUPUS

There are a few sorts of lupus; there are some lupuses that can influence the skin, for example, discoid lupus erythematosus.

Be that as it may, the term lupus is for the most part used to portray a more serious condition named fundamental lupus erythematosus additionally called SLE which influences various pieces of the body including the skin, joints just as interior organs.

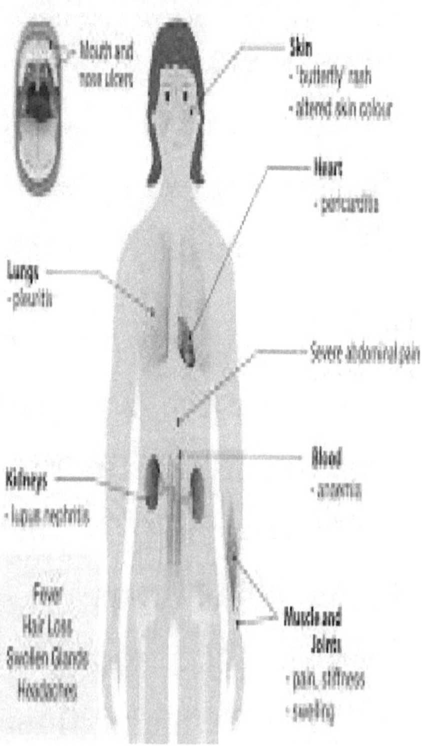

The side effects go from mellow to extreme and furthermore numerous individuals will have exceptionally significant stretches with next to zero indications before they begin encountering an unexpected erupt when the side effects are exceptionally unforgiving or serious.

People Affected By Lupus

Lupus happens in about 90% of ladies and the condition is

for the most part regular in ladies of childbearing ages that are between the age scopes of 15-50 years, nonetheless, it can likewise influence all times of people as well.

To be specific, the conditions are more uncommon in people or people of white European starting point, and are more normal in individuals or people of Africa, Caribbean or Asian cause.

CHAPTER THREE

SYMPTOMS OF LUPUS THAT ARE KNOWN

Indications of lupus can fluctuate from people to people; a few people or individuals may encounter a couple of mellow side effects while others might be harshly or seriously influenced

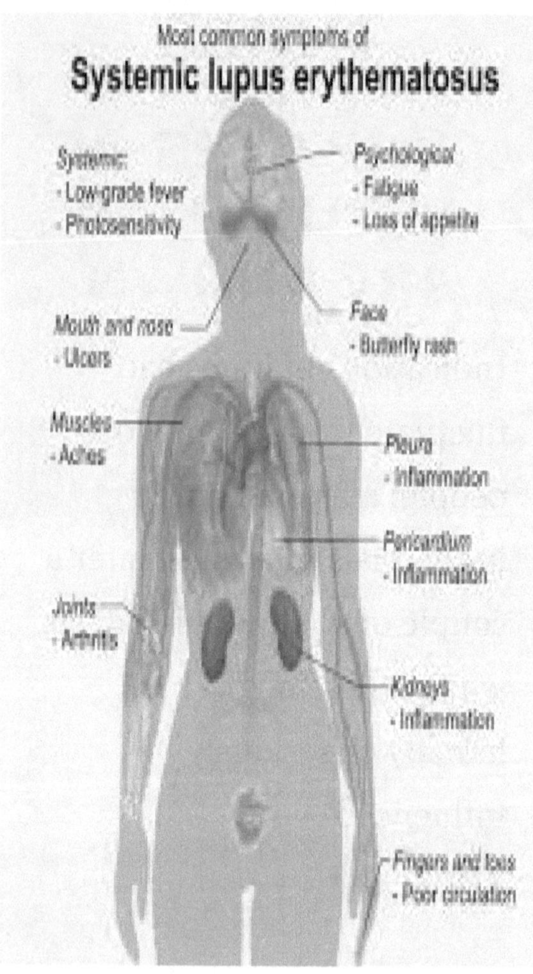

Most common symptoms of
Systemic lupus erythematosus
Systemic:
- Low-grade fever
- Photosensitivity
Psychological
- Fatigue
- Loss of appetite
Mouth and nose
- Ulcers
Face
- Butterfly rash
Muscles
- Aches
Pleura
- Inflammation
Pericardium
- Inflammation
Joints
- Arthritis
Kidneys
- Inflammation
Fingers and toes
- Poor circulation

Coming up next are side
effects of Lupus, they
include:

*Fatigue

*Joint torment

* And rashes

Exhaustion

This is one of the most
widely recognized side

effects of lupus, and you may
feel tired regardless of
whether you rested quite
well and doing ordinary
assignments, for example,
office works, and schoolwork
will make you feeling
colossally depleted.

Loads of people discover
lupus extremely troubling
just as troublesome as it
badly affects their work in
addition to public activity.

Joint Pain

For people having lupus,
they will probably encounter
joint torment in their grasp
and feet.

Furthermore, you will
understand that the agony
moves from hands to feet
just as starting with one joint
then onto the next and it
turns out to be more terrible
in the first part of the day
time.

Not at all like other sickness
that influences the joints,
lupus won't for all time harm
or distort your hands.

Rashes

Endless people with lupus
every now and again create
rashes on their skin,
generally in the face, wrists
and hands.

A rash that happens in the
over the cheeks just as the

scaffolds of the nose is extremely normal and is known as butterfly rash (or malar rash).

Rashes that are brought about by lupus show signs of improvement following a couple of days or weeks; in any case, it can keep going for a more drawn out time of or gets lasting.

Rashes that are brought about by lupus are extremely agonizing and irritated.

Furthermore, may turn out to be more regrettable on the off chance that they are presented to daylight which is named photosensitivity.

Different Symptoms of Lupus

It can likewise cause an assortment of side effects, which incorporate the accompanying:

*Shortness of breath

*Swelling of lower leg in
addition to maintenance of
liquid otherwise called
oedema

*Raynaud's wonder

; this is an ailments that
forestalls the flexibly of
blood to the hands and feet
when it turns out to be very
virus.

*Difficulty in deduction unmistakably

*Seizures

*Loss of memory

*Dry eyes

*Depression

*Chest torment

*Stomach or stomach
torment

*Headaches in addition to
headaches

*High pulse

*Loss of hair

*Regular mouth ulcers

*High temperature or fever

CHAPTER FOUR

REAL CAUSES OF LUPUS

Besides, lupus is an immune system condition, in other words, it is brought about by issues or issues in the human resistant framework.

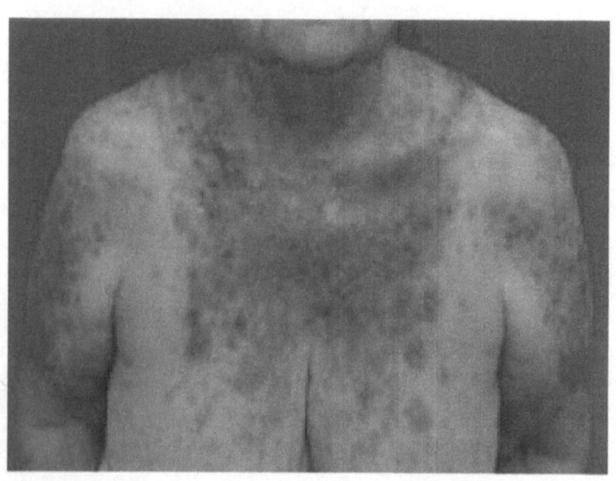

Additionally, the human safe framework assaults the normal barrier of the body against disease just as contamination, and when the invulnerable framework perceives the nearness of an irresistible body, for example, a microbes or infection all things considered. What's more, it at that point sends white platelets just as antibodies to assault it.

Coming up next are the reasons for lupus, they include:

Hereditary Factors

Here, groups of people with lupus are bound to build up the condition than different people.

There are various different hereditary transformations that makes individuals bound to create sickness or malady.

Furthermore, a hereditary transformation happens or happens when a typical guidance that was completed in specific qualities become muddled.

Ecological Factors

There are different ecological variables that are

answerable for lupus, they
are as per the following:

*Smoking

*Exposure to daylight or
natural conditions

*Changes in hormone that
happens in ladies during
pregnancy just as
pubescence

*Certain contaminations

CHAPTER FIVE

EFFICIENT DIAGNOSIS OF LUPUS

Lupus, as it is alluded to can in some cases be exceptionally hard to analyze as it has similar indications to a few other normal conditions

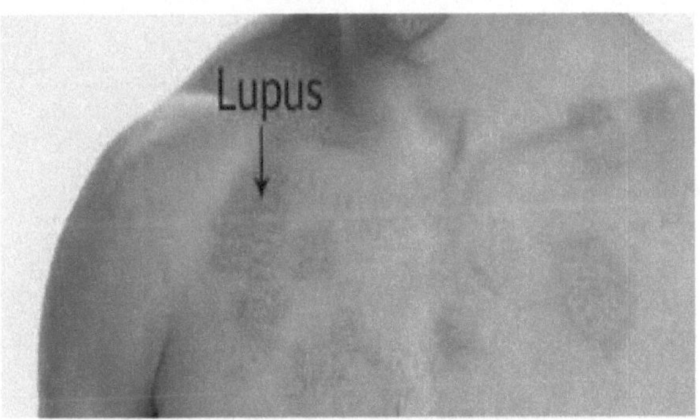

Determination can likewise be troublesome on the grounds that it varies starting with one individual then onto the next and may change every once in a while, that is there might be time when it may not be observable and there are times when it will erupt and get serious

Coming up next are approaches to analyze lupus

Blood Tests

Some blood test that might be completed incorporates

Erythrocyte Sedimentation
rate (ESR) test

This is a blood test that is
utilized to decide whether
there is irritation in your
body

This is helpful in diagnosing
SLE in light of the fact that
the condition can make
numerous zones of the body
become excited including the
joints and interior organs

This test does its capacity by
estimating how long it takes
for the red platelets to

tumble to the base of the test
tube, the quicker it falls, and
the almost certain there is an
elevated level s of irritation

Hostile to atomic immunizer
test

This test assists with
checking if there are specific
kinds of immunizer cells in
the blood known as against
atomic neutralizer

Hostile to DNA counter
acting agent test

This test assists with
checking if there are specific

sorts of antibodies in your
blood otherwise called
enemy of DNA antibodies
and on the off chance that
you have this counter acting
agent, at that point there is
an extraordinary possibility
that you have lupus

Be that as it may, the
counter acting agent is just
found in 70% of individuals
with this condition

Supplement Level Test

Supplement is a substance
that is available in the blood
that is a piece of the safe
framework, the degree of

compound might be tried to check how dynamic your lupus is

The degree of supplement in your blood decreases as the lupus turns out to be more dynamic

Other Test

When you have been determined to have lupus, you will require customary checking to perceive how the condition influences your body

On the off chance that you
have lupus, it can result to
other medical issues, for
example, kidney issues and
observing your condition
will permit the specialist to
check if any of these
inconveniences and treat
them as fast as could be
expected under the
circumstances

You may likewise need to
play out the accompanying
sweep, for example,

Automated tomography
additionally called CT
examine

Attractive reverberation
imaging additionally called
(MRI) check

Ultrasound examine

X-beam

To check whether the lupus
is influencing inside organs

CHAPTER SIX

TREATING LUPUS QUICKLY AND EFFECTIVELY

There is no solution for lupus, yet the treatment can lessen the side effects and make it exceptionally simple to live with.

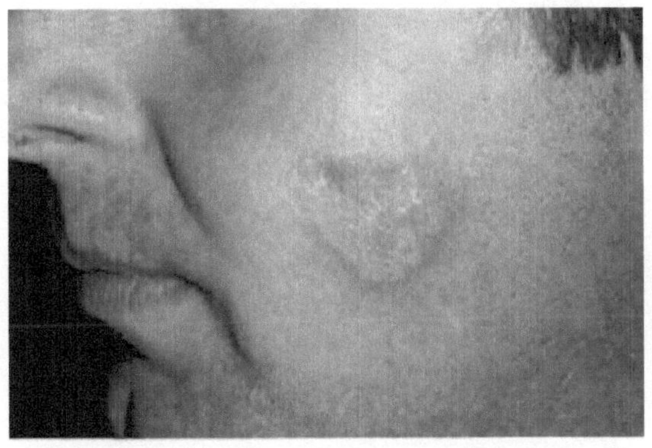

Coming up next are approaches to treat lupus

Shielding From Sunlight

Over the top introduction to daylight can most occasions make the side effects, for example, rashes exacerbate and consequently it is essential to shield yourself from the sun

This additionally incorporates wearing of garments that covers the skin, a wide cap and shades

You will likewise need to apply sunscreen with a high SPF to forestall burns from the sun

As most people get the greater part of the nutrient D from direct contact of sun on the skin, there is a higher possibility that you may not get enough nutrients because of unpredictable sun presentation and therefore you should incorporate nutrient D into your eating regimen to keep away from osteoporosis which is frail bones

Non-Steriodal Anti-Inflammatory Drugs (NSAIDs)

These are customary painkillers that help to diminish aggravation in the body, on the off chance that you are encountering joint or muscle torment because of lupus, you might be recommended NSAID to lessen the impacts

Some generally recommended NSAIDs for lupus are ibuprofen, diclofenac and naproxen

You can purchase NSAIDs,
for example, ibuprofen over
the counter if your joint
agony is gentle however for
more serious torment, you
will require a more grounded
medicine

These medications are not
appropriate for individuals
with stomach, kidney or liver
issues

Individuals with asthma
ought not ingest these
medications

Reactions

On the off chance that it is taken in extremely high portion or for an exceptionally extensive stretch of time, it can cause harm your stomach lining, which can prompt inward dying

Hydrxychloroquine

This is a medication that is utilized to treat jungle fever, yet it is likewise viable in treating a portion of the indications of lupus, for example, joint and muscle torment, rashes and exhaustion

You should take this medication for between 6-12 weeks to see the advantages

Symptoms

The symptoms of this medications are remarkable and may incorporate acid reflux, looseness of the bowels, rashes and cerebral pain

Cortiocosteriods

This is a sort of medication that assists with lessening irritation quick, they are likewise compelling in

treating lupus, however are
recommended if the
condition is extreme

Symptoms

At the point when this
medication is recommended,
it is normally given in little
portion since high dosages of
corticosteroids can prompt
destructive reactions

They incorporate

*High pulse

*gaining of weight

*Thinning of your skin

*thinning of your bone

These medications are
protected and viable sort of
treatment

Immunosuppressants

These are sort of medication
that assists with stifling your
safe framework, they help to
improve your indications of
lupus by assisting with
constraining the harm your
invulnerable framework

causes when assaults sound
pieces of the body

Normally recommended
immunosuppressant's
medications incorporate
azathioprine, methotrexate,
mycophenolate mofetil, and
cyclophosphamide

Reactions

These drug are possibly
recommended in the event
that you have serious lupus

This is on the grounds that
this medication is amazing

and can cause symptoms, for
example,

Expanded danger of disease

Liver harm

Weight gain

Abundance hair
development

Skin break out

Migraine

Fast dying

Swollen gums

The runs

Regurgitating

Loss of hunger

These medications can
likewise cause birth
absconds in the event that
they are taken during
pregnancy

Danger of Infection

Taking immunosuppressant
can build the danger of
building up a disease

The side effects of
contamination may in some
cases take after those of
cutting edge lupus, for
example,

High fever

Hack

Consuming sensation while
peeing

Hack

Fever

You ought to likewise
abstain from reaching those
with contamination

Rituximab

This is another sort of
medicine that is utilized in
individuals with extreme
lupus that don't react to
different medicines

It was initially intended to
treat particular kinds of

malignancy, for example,
lymphoma however has been
demonstrated to treat
various immune system
ailments, for example, lupus
and joint pain

It works by holding and
slaughtering cells called B
cells which are liable for
creating antibodies that
cause lupus

It is controlled legitimately
to the vein

Symptoms

The normal symptoms of
rituximab incorporate

Heaving

Discombobulation

Influenza like side effects,
for example, high
temperature

Belimumab

This is a prescription that is
given to individuals with
lupus that reacts to different
medicines

It accomplishes its work by
official to development
factors that encourages the
B-cells to endure

It is managed
straightforwardly to the
veins for a long time called
mixture

The initial three dosages are
given 14 days separated and
the prescription is allowed
once per month

The End